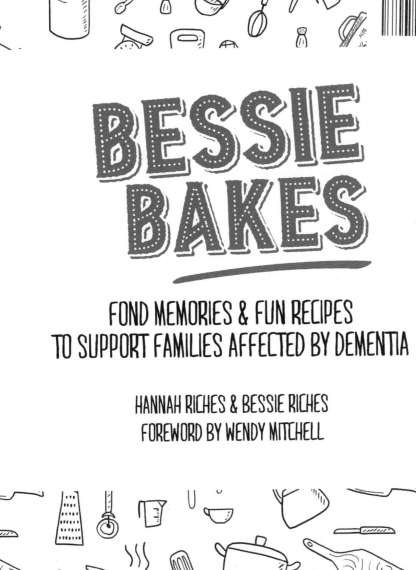

BESSIE BAKES

FOND MEMORIES & FUN RECIPES
TO SUPPORT FAMILIES AFFECTED BY DEMENTIA

HANNAH RICHES & BESSIE RICHES

FOREWORD BY WENDY MITCHELL

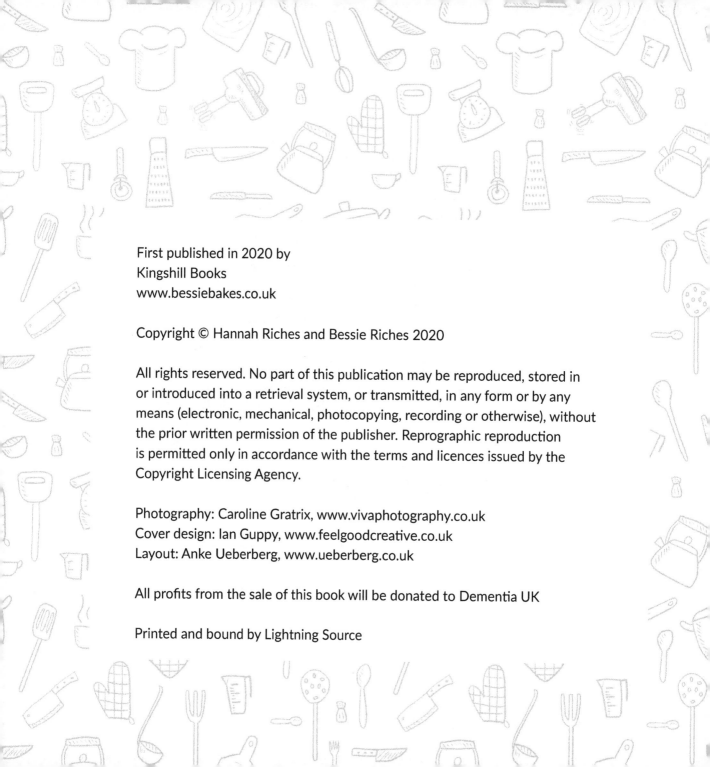

For my Daddy, Neil

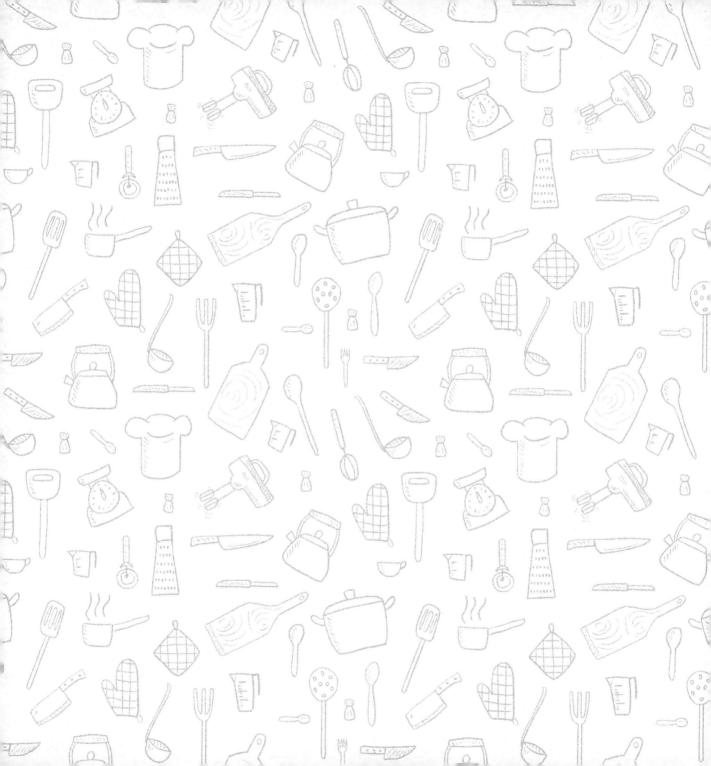

Contents

Foreword

There's nothing like the smell of freshly baked cake fresh from the oven; we all have our favourite. I used to bake every weekend. When Hannah asked me if I had a favourite recipe from the past, there could only be one, as my daughters, as small children, loved my Orange Cake. Tiny fingers, tucking into a tiny slice, crumbs being rescued from wherever they fell.

Sadly I now live with dementia in tow, having been diagnosed in 2014. My ability to bake faded as soon as dementia took hold. However, now my recipe, along with many others, has been collected and baked by Hannah's daughter, Bessie, to raise money for Dementia UK, who provide specialist dementia support for families through their Admiral Nurse service. I and my daughters would benefit greatly from the comfort of having an Admiral Nurse, but sadly they're in very short supply.

Thank you, Bessie, for keeping those baking memories alive as our memories fade and, in doing so, raising much-needed funds for a wonderful charity.

Wendy Mitchell

Author of the *Sunday Times* bestseller
Somebody I Used to Know

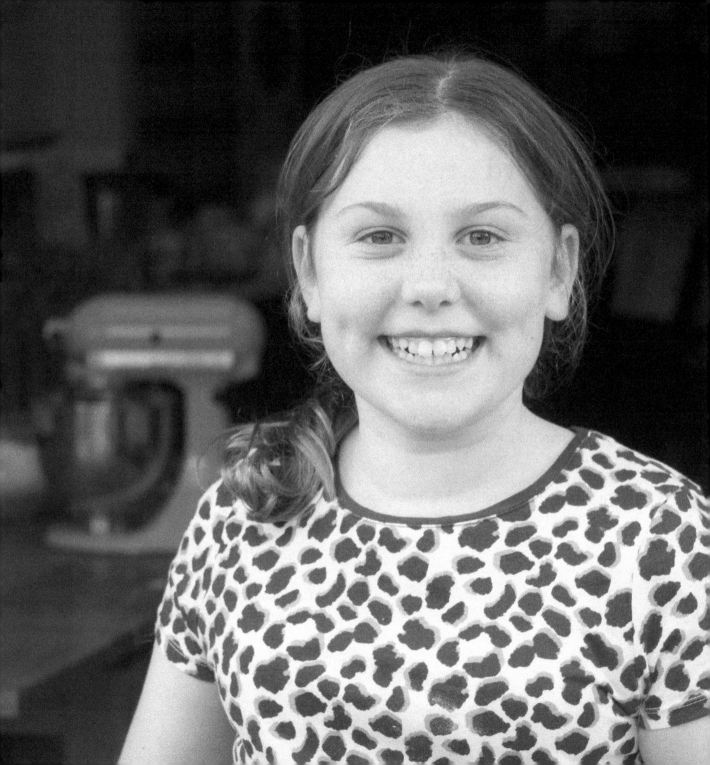

Hello from Bessie

I am Bessie. I decided to make this cookbook to raise money for a charity that is awfully close to my heart, Dementia UK. This is because my daddy has dementia. He got it when I was 5.

I have done lots already for this charity, like dementia sales and a coffee morning. I do them with one of my best friends, Mariella, and her sister Cora. I have lots of fun doing the sales and always look forward to them. But because of Covid-19 we have obviously not been able to do them.

I was trying to think of ideas to raise money, and my mum and I had this idea of a dementia cookbook, because my favourite thing to do is bake. I emailed lots of friends and family and asked for recipes that have good memories for them, and I had loads of replies!

I have tried all the dishes, cakes, biscuits and other treats in this book. They were all sooo good, and I really hope that you have fun trying out these recipes.

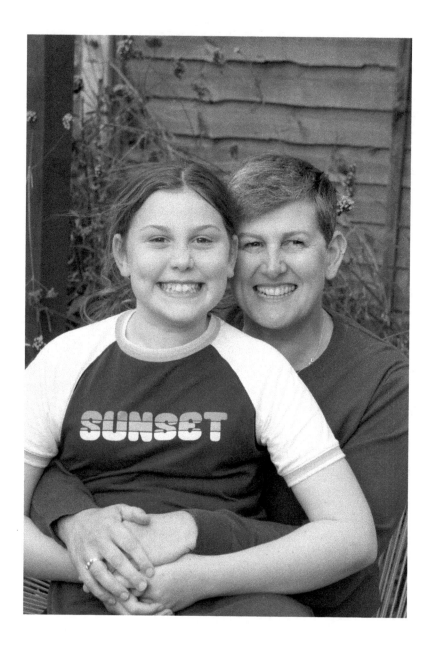

Introduction

My grandmother was an amazing baker, and it was always a treat to sneak a peak into the biscuit tin as a young child. She passed down a love of baking (and eating) to all of her nine grandchildren. Bessie and I recently flicked through her handwritten recipe book, which she started in 1976. It was a trip down Memory Lane for me, and interesting for Bessie to see some of the original recipes that my cousins had sent to her. I love how they are all attributed to friends and family members: Lesley's Chocolate Refrigerator Cake, Grandpa Dixon's Green Tomato Chutney, Duncombe Biscuits...

With Bessie's permission I have included quite a few recipes from my grandmother's repertoire, as the extended family still bake her cakes and biscuits on a regular basis.

Having started this project, I found it interesting that all my favourite family recipes are sweet, whereas my husband's are all savoury. He loved to cook and had a handful of favourites that his mother had taught him. His father managed Bernie Inns, and his mother used to cook for their events. There was Swedish Chicken, Mexican Rice Chicken and Toad in the Hole with Onion Gravy. Sadly Neil can't remember the recipes or cook them anymore, and they weren't written down.

The girls don't remember Daddy cooking but it was a big love of his, and I am pleased that he has passed it on to Bessie. During lockdown, when he was finding things tough with his routine all out of whack, Lizzie, our Admiral Nurse, suggested that Bess and Neil should bake together. It was a fabulous idea, and they had some lovely mornings making cookies. It's fair to say they also enjoyed having a cup of tea and tasting the fruits of their labours afterwards.

In order to keep Bessie occupied over the school holidays, I suggested she contact family and friends and ask them to send her their favourite recipes and let her know why they were special. Food can be an amazing way to connect with others, and we have loved reading all their emails and trying out the recipes. Unsurprisingly, we are not the only family to have a sweet tooth, but we have some savoury treats too.

The original idea was for Bessie to make the food, then write up the recipe; but I guess no one will be surprised that the project morphed into me doing the writing. I have included her comments where appropriate.

Thank you for supporting us by buying the book. We hope you find something to enjoy with your family.

Hannah

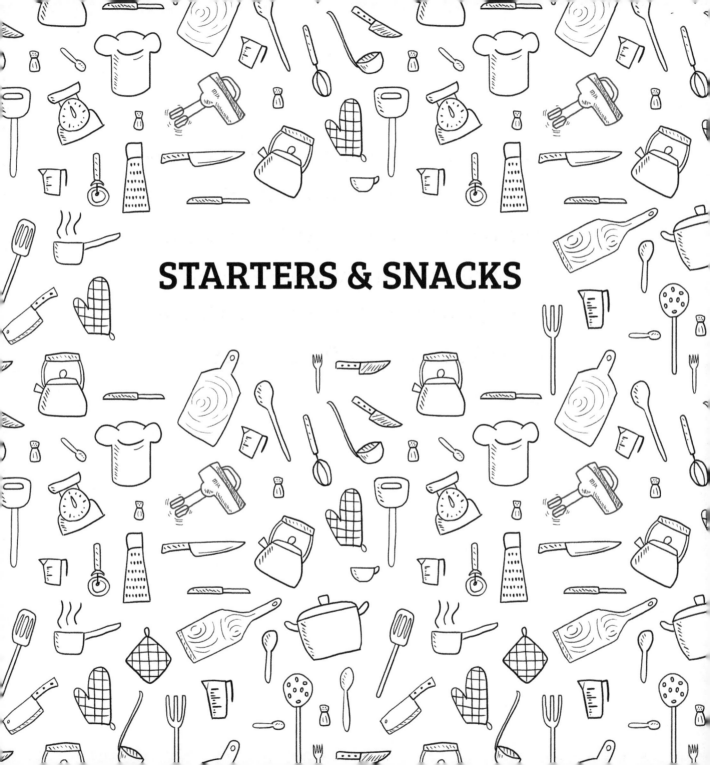

STARTERS & SNACKS

"These are really simple and fun to make. Bessie has made them loads this summer and is now an expert. Neil liked them so much he ate a whole plateful left on the side, and Bessie had to quickly make a new batch in time for a lunch with friends."

Hannah

Bessie's Cheese Straws

YOU WILL NEED...

ready-rolled puff pastry at
    room temperature
Cheddar cheese, grated
Parmesan cheese
1 egg, beaten

MAKE IT!

1. Preheat the oven to 200°, 180° (fan), gas mark 6, and line a baking sheet with greaseproof paper. Carefully unroll the puff pastry.
2. Sprinkle the grated cheese evenly over the puff pastry, then fold in half so that the cheese is inside. Lightly roll the pastry a couple of times to gently squash the cheese into the pastry.
3. Cut into 2cm strips – we use a pizza cutter for ease, but a sharp knife will do. Twist these strips 3–4 times, then place on the baking sheet and brush with the beaten egg. Place into the hot oven for 20 minutes until golden and crunchy.
4. Leave to cool and serve with hummus or homemade tzatziki for a really tasty snack.

Bessie's Top Tip

Use a nice strong cheddar for the best flavour, and don't leave these out unattended – or they may disappear!

9

"My girls are not great at eating cooked vegetables but demolish this, so I serve it a lot. Our summer favourite is having it alongside a roast chicken and homemade chips. Bessie was reluctant to include the recipe because she didn't want to divulge the family secret, but she relented when I reminded her the whole point of this cookbook was to share family recipes. So shhh – try this coleslaw but don't tell Bess!"

Hannah

Aunty Wendy's Coleslaw

YOU WILL NEED...

green cabbage
a red onion
2 carrots
half a lemon
mayonnaise

MAKE IT!

1. Finely chop the cabbage and the red onion. Grate the carrots.
2. Put all the veg into a large bowl and squeeze the lemon juice over the top.
3. Add a large dollop of mayonnaise and mix it all together. Season to taste.

Bessie's Top Tip

I don't like a lot of mayonnaise but my sister does – just adjust to your taste.

"Eating together has always been important in my family – my dad was famous for his Ueberberg breakfasts. This dish has been a regular at parties and summer barbecues, and at our Christmas meat fondue dinner, for many years. My dad in particular loved it, simply eaten with 'peely' potatoes."

Anke

Tzatziki

YOU WILL NEED...

1kg Greek yoghurt
   (full fat is best)
1½–2 cucumbers
3 cloves garlic (more if
   you like it spicier)
a handful of mint leaves
salt and pepper

MAKE IT!

1. Wash and coarsely grate the cucumber (leave the skin on) into a big sieve or colander set over a bowl. The grated cucumber can be left to drain while you get on with preparing the yoghurt.

2. Put the yoghurt in a suitably sized bowl. Peel the garlic cloves and put through the garlic press. Slice the mint leaves thinly. Stir garlic, mint leaves and a generous pinch of salt into the yoghurt.

3. Now, with clean hands, squeeze as much of the water out of the grated cucumber as you can, until there's hardly any liquid seeping out between your fingers.

4. Tip the cucumber into the yoghurt, stir through and season to taste with more salt and a grind of pepper if you think it needs it. This will keep for 2–3 days in the fridge (if it lasts that long!)

Bessie's Top Tip

Oh my gosh, I loved this. We ate it with fajitas and then with grilled chicken the following day.

"I love this recipe. I do it a lot and know it off by heart. It never fails – in fact when my friend Joe comes round we nearly always have it because we are both obsessed with it."

Bessie

Bessie & Joe's Nachos

YOU WILL NEED...

1 pack of cool original
   Doritos
Cheddar cheese (as much as
   you like, I use quite a lot)
homemade salsa (see below)
   or if you're really hungry
   use a jar from the shop
other toppings (optional):
   guacamole or the tzatziki
   go well with this

MAKE IT!

1. Empty the pack of Doritos into a large, oven-safe bowl. Spoon the salsa on the Doritos.
2. Add other toppings if you would like them. You could always serve these on the side so fussy people don't moan.
3. Now grate the amount of cheese you would like and sprinkle it all over the Doritos and salsa.
4. Place under the grill at a high heat for two minutes or until the cheese has melted. Put the bowl on the table and share with your friends.

Bessie's Top Tip
Use 2 packs of Doritos if feeding more than 4 people, and of course you can use any flavour.

Bessie's Homemade Salsa

YOU WILL NEED...

2 big tomatoes
6 little tomatoes (baby plum
   or cherry)
1 red onion
a glug of white wine vinegar
half a lime
mixed herbs
salt and pepper

MAKE IT!

1. Finely chop the tomatoes and the onion.
2. Put both into a bowl and add the juice of the lime, a sprinkle of mixed herbs and the vinegar. Season.

Bessie's Top Tip
My mum suggests adding some fresh coriander and a glug of olive oil, but I don't think it needs it.

15

"Mexican food is our go-to family comfort food and this has been eaten on countless significant occasions. You can be flexible with the recipe and it still tastes good."

Aunty Emma

Aunty Emma's Guacamole

YOU WILL NEED...

3–4 ripe avocados
4–6 spring onions
juice of 1 lime, or to taste
a few drops of Tabasco sauce
   (optional)
2–3 garlic cloves, crushed
salt and pepper
1 tablespoon chopped fresh
   coriander (or more, to
   taste)

MAKE IT!

1. Finely chop the onion and mash the avocado with a fork.
2. Add lime juice, garlic and Tabasco and mix. Season and sprinkle with coriander.
3. Serve with a big bag of tortillas, tacos and fresh veg sticks.

Bessie's Top Tip

Try this with my nachos!
If you're not using the guacamole immediately, bury one of the avocado stones in it to prevent discolouring.

"My mother made smoked mackerel pate every year as the starter for Christmas Day. I am sure it is very tasty on other days of the year, but to me it says Christmas. I used to help her prepare this – she served it with slices of toast cut into triangles, shredded iceberg lettuce and a slice of lemon. I have been known to have it in a sandwich as a welcome alternative to turkey on Boxing Day."

Hannah

Grandma Lesley's Smoked Mackerel Pate

YOU WILL NEED...
250g smoked mackerel
180g tub of cream cheese
juice of half a lemon
salt and pepper

MAKE IT!
1. Place all ingredients into a bowl and use a stick blender to mush together.
2. Serve in a pretty bowl with toast, a slice of lemon and a garnish of lettuce.

Bessie's Top Tip
Be careful with the stick blender – Aunty Jo once took the top off her finger using hers and now Mummy warns us about this whenever we use it!

"I have been making this for years but when the shops ran out of yeast during the lockdown it was a really useful alternative. And it's really fun for kids to have a go."

Amanda

Flatbread

YOU WILL NEED...
300g self-raising flour
300g natural yoghurt
1 teaspoon baking powder

MAKE IT!
1. Mix flour and baking powder. Put the yoghurt into a bowl and slowly add the flour, stirring with a fork or wooden spoon, until it comes together.
2. Turn out onto a lightly floured surface and knead for a few minutes until it forms a soft, elastic dough.
3. Cut the dough into golfball-sized pieces. Roll out each piece to about 3mm in thickness.
4. Heat a non-stick frying pan and dry-fry each flatbread for 20–30 seconds each side.

Bessie's Top Tip
Make this to go with the falafel and tzatziki or balti chicken. You get pretty sticky but it is fun!

"One of my favourite savoury foods is falafel. I was taught how to make it by a friend who is from Iraq, and a big part of her culture is spending time cooking with family and friends, so she likes to teach me new recipes. As this is passed from person to person there are no precise measurements!"

Fiona

Falafel

YOU WILL NEED...

lots of chickpeas (soaked
    for 12 hours and then
    cooked on a very low heat
    overnight in slow cooker)
a couple of cloves of garlic
lots and lots of fresh
    coriander and parsley
1 teaspoon of bicarbonate of
    soda
1 onion
a pinch of cumin
oil, to cook

MAKE IT!

1. Blend everything together with a stick blender or food processor. It will end as a green mixture.
2. Chill in the fridge for a bit: this makes it easier to roll the mixture into golfball-sized balls.
3. Fry in oil, a couple at a time. Any leftover mixture freezes well for another quick tea.
4. Serve with pitta, hummus or tahini sauce, and salad.

Bessie's Top Tip

We used two tins of chickpeas so didn't need to soak and cook them overnight. I served these with Anke's tzatziki and homemade flatbread. I won't lie – they are not my favourite* but my mum *loved* them.

....

*   Hannah says, 'When the girls were little I taught them to
say "Thank you, but it's not my favourite" if they didn't like
something they were served at a friend's house and wanted
to leave it. Much nicer than "Urgh, I hate that!" It must have
sunk in.'

23

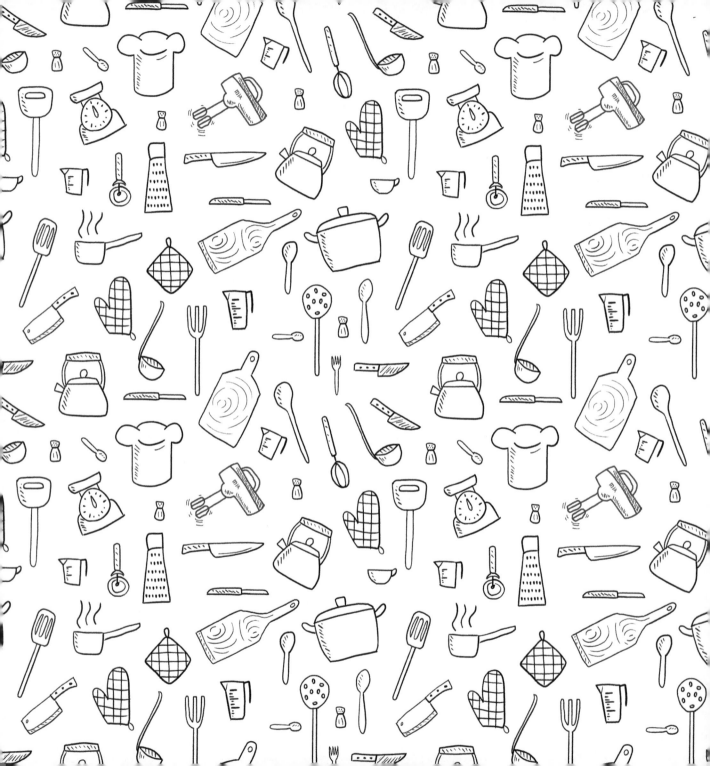

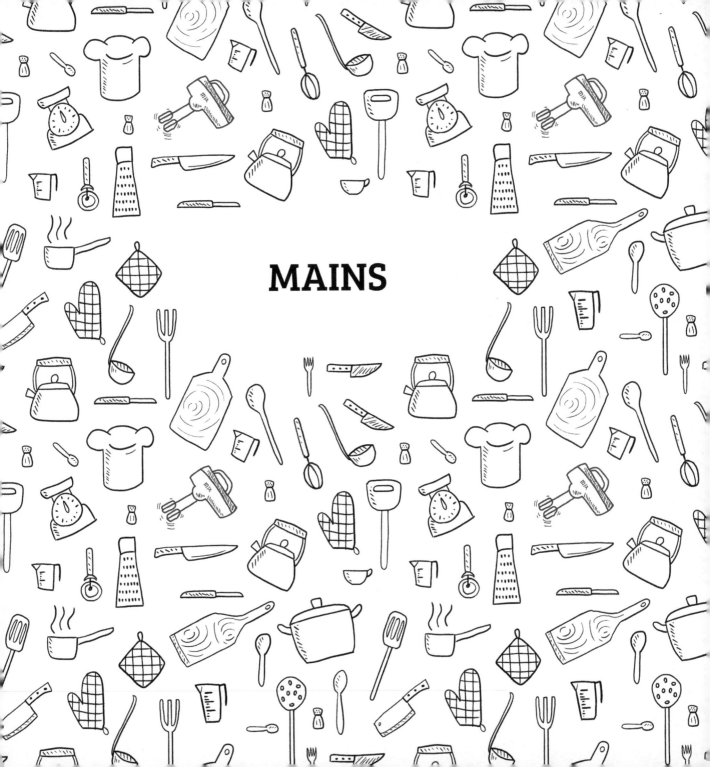

MAINS

"Our friend Amanda's mum, Shirley, passed this on to her daughters, and we are delighted that Amanda and her kids have passed it on to us – it's become a family favourite!"

Hannah

Oven-roasted Tomato Sauce

YOU WILL NEED...

2kg ripe tomatoes

2 big onions

12 garlic cloves

4 tablespoons olive oil

2 tablespoons balsamic
vinegar

1 tablespoon sugar

½ teaspoon sea salt

½ teaspoon freshly ground
black pepper

MAKE IT!

1. Preheat the oven to 200°, 180° (fan), gas mark 6. Cut tomatoes in half and arrange on a big baking tray.

2. Scatter with onions and garlic, drizzle with olive oil and toss. Bake for 1 hour or until the tomatoes are soft and slightly scorched, and the onions are cooked. Remove from the oven and cool for 30 minutes.

3. Fish out the garlic cloves, squeeze the cooked garlic from each one and discard the skins. Put into a bowl and add balsamic vinegar, sugar, salt and pepper.

4. Either simply stir with a wooden spoon until you have a thick and lumpy sauce or whizz briefly with a stick blender or in the food processor until thick and smooth.

5. Use about 500ml to serve 4 with pasta: reheat in a saucepan and season to taste with salt and pepper. Also good as a base on homemade pizza.

Bessie's Top Tip

We crumbled some feta cheese on the pasta and sauce – it was very good.

27

"Amanda and I met at university in Birmingham over 25 years ago and have shared many drunken baltis together. After uni I joined the West Midlands Police and continued to enjoy the local cuisine, often with Neil and friends. He always ordered a chicken and mushroom balti so when cooking Manda's recipe I would definitely add mushrooms. I don't have a wood oven so authentic naan bread is out, but you could try the yoghurt flatbread."

Hannah

Sweet and Sour Chicken and Mushroom Balti

YOU WILL NEED...

650g skinned and cubed
  chicken (breast or thigh)
6 tablespoons tomato puree
4 tablespoons Greek yoghurt
4 tablespoons mango
  chutney
1½ teaspoons garam masala
1 garlic clove, crushed
1 teaspoon salt
1 teaspoon chili powder
4 tablespoons oil
¼ pint (120ml) water
2 fresh green chillies,
  chopped
2 tablespoons fresh
  coriander, chopped
2 tablespoons single cream

MAKE IT!

1. Put the tomato puree and Greek yoghurt into a bowl. Add the garam masala, chilli powder, garlic, mango chutney and salt and stir until thoroughly mixed.

2. Heat the oil in a deep frying pan or large karahi. Turn down the heat and add the yoghurt and spice mixture. Bring to the boil and cook for 2 minutes, stirring occasionally.

3. Add the chicken pieces and stir until they are well coated. Add the water to thin the sauce slightly. Continue cooking for 5–7 minutes or until the chicken is tender. Add mushrooms halfway through.

4. Add half the green chillies, half the coriander and the cream and cook for a further 2 minutes. Check that the chicken is cooked through.

5. Transfer to a warmed dish and garnish with the remaining chillies and coriander.

"I got really annoyed when I realised I hadn't asked Mum to write down any of her recipes – all those classics gone. Such a crime. Swedish Chicken was a family favourite: great in the summer and especially good as a late-night snack."

Adam

Granny Shelagh's 'Swedish' Chicken

YOU WILL NEED...

cold cooked chicken, chopped into chunks

cold cooked rice

1 banana, sliced

1 apple, cored and cut into chunks

a handful of grapes, halved

1 stick of celery, sliced

very large dollop of mayonnaise

a sprinkle of curry powder (optional)

MAKE IT!

1. OK – its pretty simple: mix all ingredients together in a big bowl and season to taste.

2. Leave to chill in the fridge for 30 minutes. This only really keeps until the bananas start to go brown, so make a big portion and demolish it fast.

Bessie's Top Tip

Leave out the banana!

66This is one of my cousin Jo's (Aunty Jo to Bessie and Milly) go-to easy supper dishes. Her two sons play American Football and have hearty appetites so they wolf through this very quickly. We have made this quite a few times and it is now firmly ensconced in our family repertoire, although my inept plaiting skills never fail to provide amusement to the girls.99

Hannah

Aunty Jo's Sausage Plait

YOU WILL NEED...

1 pack of puff pastry
1 pack of sausage meat
1 pack of sage and onion
   stuffing mix
1 egg, beaten

MAKE IT!

1. Preheat oven to 200°, 180° (fan), gas mark 6. Take the puff pastry out of fridge and let it come to room temperature. Make up the stuffing mix as per the pack instructions and leave to cool.

2. Put the sausage meat and stuffing mix into a bowl and mix together – go on, get messy and use your (clean) hands!

3. Carefully unroll ready-rolled puff pastry (if in a block, use a rolling pin to roll into a rectangle about 3–4mm thick) and transfer it to a baking sheet lined with baking paper.

4. Place the sausage meat and stuffing mixture in a fat sausage shape lengthways down the centre of the pastry rectangle, leaving a gap of about 3cm from the top and bottom and 5cm from the sides.

5. Now the fun part – plaiting time! Cut a diagonal line from the top corner of the sausage mix out to the edge of the pastry. Repeat at 2cm intervals down one side and do the same on the other. Brush these strips with beaten egg. Now fold the top pastry piece up onto the top end of the sausage mix, then fold over the first left-hand side pastry strip and repeat with the first right-hand strip. Carry on, alternating left and right strips to cover the sausage mix with a pastry plait.

6. Brush with egg and put into the preheated oven for 45–60 minutes until golden and cooked through. Cut into slices and serve.

"Every Christmas Eve we go over to Bessie's godmother Caz's house near Marlow. Ian cooks us his fish pie, and his son Will bakes a chocolate log. Bessie and Milly are not massive fans of the fish pie, but they eat it all up so they can have the chocolate log! Then we go on a walk – of which they are also not fans. Gotta love family traditions!"

Hannah

Ian's Christmas Eve Fish Pie

YOU WILL NEED...

5 large potatoes, peeled and
  cut into 2.5cm cubes
salt and freshly ground black
  pepper
2 large handfuls of spinach
1 onion, finely chopped
extra olive oil
about 285ml double cream
2 good handfuls of grated
  Cheddar or Parmesan
juice of one lemon
1 heaped teaspoon of
  English mustard
1 large handful of flat leaf
  parsley, finely chopped
445g haddock or cod fillets,
  skin removed and sliced
  into strips
nutmeg (optional)

MAKE IT!

1. Preheat oven to 230°, 210° (fan), gas mark 8. Put potatoes into salted boiling water, bring back to the boil and boil for 2 minutes.

2. Steam the spinach in a colander over the pan; this will only take 1 minute. When the spinach has collapsed, remove from colander and gently squeeze out excess moisture. Then drain and mash the cooked potatoes – add a bit of olive oil, salt, pepper, and a touch of nutmeg if you like.

3. In a separate pan, fry the onion and carrot in a little olive oil over a medium heat for about 5 minutes, then add double cream and bring to the boil. Remove from the heat and add the cheese, lemon juice, mustard, and parsley.

4. Put the spinach and fish into an appropriately sized dish and mix, pouring over the creamy vegetable sauce. Spread the mashed potato on top of the fish.

5. Place in the oven for about 25–30 minutes until the potatoes are golden, then admire your creation before it all gets gobbled up.

Bessie's Top Tip

Why not leave out the spinach so your kids don't have to pick it out? I wouldn't say no to some frozen peas as a side order with this.

"When my mother died, we all thought my father would end up surviving on white crusty bread slathered in butter, and Chelsea buns. Actually he coped OK and became a fan of the slow cooker, so on Sundays when we visited, he often made this casserole. It also became his contribution at the annual cousins' gathering."

Hannah

Babar's Italian Chicken Casserole

YOU WILL NEED...

3 chicken breasts
1 onion, chopped
2 carrots, sliced
2 celery stalks, sliced
¼ bottle white wine
240ml chicken stock
a handful of mushrooms
  (optional)
Italian mixed herbs
2 bay leaves
salt and pepper

MAKE IT!

1. Put the onions, celery and carrots into the bottom of the slow cooker and layer the chicken breasts and mushrooms (if you don't have fussy kids) on top.
2. Prepare the chicken stock, add a pinch of herbs and add to the slow cooker. Finally pour white wine over the veg and chicken and add the bay leaves.
3. Put on the lid and cook on a low setting for 8 hours. This should be plenty of time but check the chicken is cooked through before serving.

Hannah's Top Tip

I am sure it could be cooked on a low heat in the oven, where you could also throw in a couple of jacket potatoes to accompany it.

"Here is a recipe that was a real family favourite and reminds me and my three sisters of our mum. Mum always served it with 'duchess potatoes' – posh mash, piped into swirls and browned in the oven. My Dad developed dementia a few years after my mum died but he continued to enjoy his food – especially this dish, and chocolate ginger."

Jo

Jo & Sisters' Chicken Casserole

YOU WILL NEED...

3 chicken breasts

1 onion

2 leeks

2 sticks celery

2 carrots

about 500ml chicken stock

200g mushrooms, sliced

25g butter

1 tablespoon olive oil

1 tablespoon plain flour

a little cream if desired, for a
    richer sauce

MAKE IT!

1. Chop all of the veg except the mushrooms and put in a saucepan with the whole chicken breasts.

2. Cover with chicken stock and simmer for 45 minutes. Remove the chicken and cut into bite sized pieces.

3. Reduce the chicken stock if necessary, so you are left with about 150ml.

4. Fry the mushrooms in a large pan in the butter and olive oil until slightly brown, then stir in the flour and cook gently, stirring all the time. Gradually add the chicken stock to make a thick sauce.

5. Finally, add the cooked chicken and veg and stir in the cream. Heat through and serve.

Bessie's Top Tip

Posh mash is fun to make!

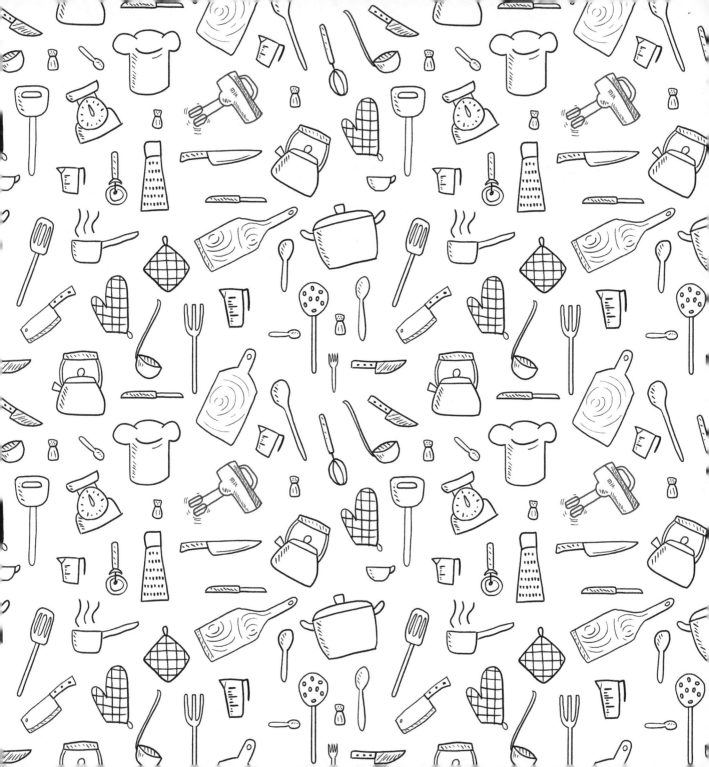

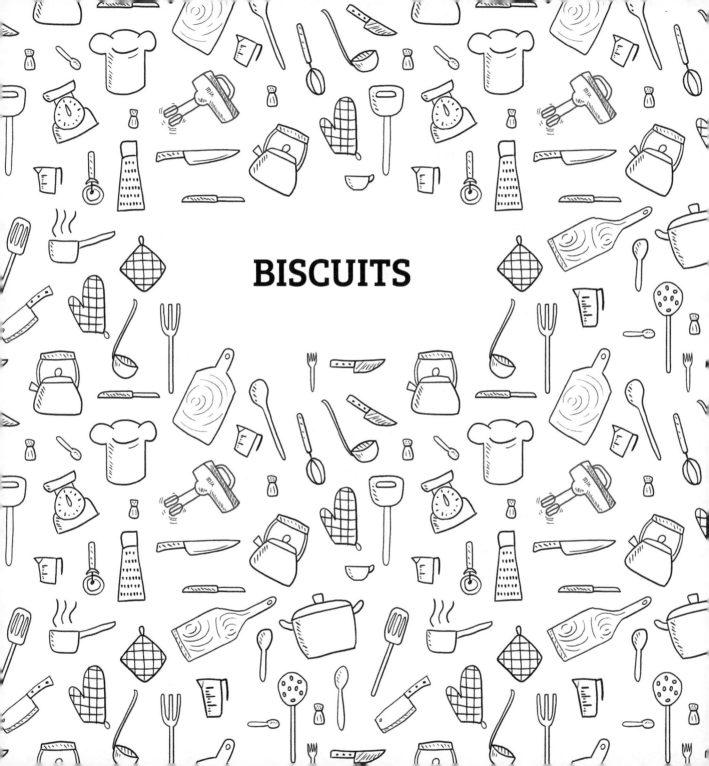

BISCUITS

"Grandma Joy was an excellent baker, and she always had fresh cake or homemade biscuits in the tin. However, if you ever dared to eat these straight from the tin you got into big trouble! No – there always had to be a tray, a tray cloth, tea served from a teapot into a bone china cup-and-saucer, and biscuits served on a plate. No exception! But when biscuits taste this good, maybe they deserve the ceremony."

Hannah

Duncombe Biscuits

YOU WILL NEED...

170g porridge oats
170g granulated sugar
85g plain flour
1 teaspoon ground ginger
140g Stork margarine
1 tablespoon syrup
1 teaspoon bicarbonate of
  soda
about 2 tablespoons warm
  water

MAKE IT!

1. Preheat the oven to 180°, 160° (fan), gas mark 4.
2. In a bowl, mix sugar, oats, flour and ground ginger.
3. Put margarine and syrup into a pan and gently heat until the margarine melts, then add to the oat-and-flour mixture in bowl.
4. Mix bicarbonate of soda with warm water, stir into the biscuit mixture and let cool for few minutes.
5. Put large teaspoons of the mixture onto a greased baking tray and place in the oven for about 20–25 minutes.
6. Remove from the oven and cut into squares if the biscuits have joined up or leave if OK. Lift with a knife or spatula onto a tray to cool. They set very quickly, so remove them before they set hard!

"For my 11th birthday my parents bought me a session called Cooking It. You can take home what you have made and share it with your family. I remember looking at the packets of Oreos and wishing I could just eat all of them there and then. My family loved these biscuits so we asked for the recipe, and I haven't stopped making them since. The Oreo practically melts into the vanilla biscuit, and that is definitely my favourite part about it."

Luke

Oreo Chocolate Chip Cookies

YOU WILL NEED...

220g softened butter
100g light brown sugar
80g golden caster sugar
1 large egg
1 tablespoon vanilla extract
400g plain flour
½ teaspoon salt
1 teaspoon baking powder
140g chocolate chips

NB Don't double this recipe, it makes a lot!

MAKE IT!

1. Preheat oven to 200°, 180° (fan), gas mark 6.
2. Cream butter and sugars, and then add the egg and vanilla. Mix well until combined.
3. In a separate bowl, mix the flour, salt and baking powder. Slowly add to the wet ingredients, one tablespoon at a time, until well combined. Then stir in the chocolate chips.
4. Grease two baking trays. Take a scoop of your cookie mix and flatten. Place an Oreo biscuit in the middle of the cookie dough, and then place an equal amount of cookie dough on top.
5. Seal all of the edges by pinching your thumbs together. Repeat with the remainder of the dough.
6. Finally, sprinkle a pinch of sea salt on top of every cookie.
7. Put the trays in the preheated oven and bake for 9–13 minutes until golden brown. Cool on a wire rack.

Bessie's Top Tip

We made a few of these and froze the leftover cookie dough: we crumbled the Oreo biscuits into chunks and mixed them into the dough, then rolled the dough into balls just smaller than a golfball and put them in the freezer, to cook from frozen when friends come round.

"My mum's favourite biscuits are 'diggers' or Anzac Biscuits. Anzac biscuits were originally called soldier's biscuits, and 'digger' is slang for 'soldier' in Australia and New Zealand. The recipe came from a PTA cookbook to raise funds for my primary school, sometime in the late 1970s. My mum has been making them for over 40 years!"

Fiona

Digger Biscuits

YOU WILL NEED...

125g self-raising flour

125g rolled oats

85g desiccated coconut

60g milk powder

85g sugar

2 tablespoons of syrup or
  honey

125g butter

1½ teaspoons of bicarbonate
  of soda

2 tablespoons of boiling
  water

MAKE IT!

1. Mix together oats, flour, sugar, coconut and milk.
2. Melt syrup and butter. Mix bicarb and water and add to the melted mixture. Mix with the dry ingredients.
3. Place heaped teaspoon onto greased trays, allowing room to spread.
4. Bake at 180°, 160° (fan), gas mark 4 for about 20 minutes.

Bessie's Top Tip

These are great for taking on camping trips – Fiona always brings a huge tin of diggers along to our annual Salcombe camping weekend.

47

These are my favourite homemade biscuits. I make them with raisins or sultanas, and add the juice of the orange too. Very tasty.

George

George's Shrewsbury Biscuits

YOU WILL NEED...

125g butter or block
   margarine
150g caster sugar
2 egg yolks
225g plain flour
rind of lemon or orange,
   grated
50g raisins or sultanas

MAKE IT!

1. Preheat the oven to 180°, 160° (fan), gas mark 4, and grease two baking sheets.
2. Cream butter and sugar together until pale and fluffy. Add the egg yolks and beat well.
3. Stir in the flour and grated lemon rind and mix to a fairly firm dough with a round-bladed knife.
4. Place the dough on a lightly floured surface and knead lightly.
5. Roll out to about 5mm thick. Cut into rounds with a 6cm fluted biscuit cutter and place on the baking sheets.
6. Bake in the oven for about 15 minutes until firm and a very light brown colour.

Bessie's Top Tip

I made these for my Dad's old army buddies when they visited – they loved them.

49

"You may know this as millionaire's shortbread, but to anyone in our family this is Wellington Square – no one seems to know why. Grandma made this every Christmas or on demand for a pleading grandchild. This takes a bit of time so it's not often made nowadays, but it's definitely worth the effort."

Hannah

Wellington Square

YOU WILL NEED...

115g plain flour
60g semolina
60g caster sugar
a pinch of salt
115g butter

115g margarine
115g soft brown sugar
2 level tablespoon golden
   syrup
1 small can condensed milk
a few drops vanilla essence

150g plain chocolate

MAKE IT!

1. Preheat the oven to 180°, 160° (fan), gas mark 4. Grease and line a 18 x 18cm shallow tin with baking paper.

2. Sift flour, semolina and salt into a mixing bowl and stir in the sugar and salt. Cut the butter into small pieces and rub in using your fingertips, then knead mixture to a dough.

3. Press into the base of a tin, levelling surface as much as possible. Bake on the centre shelf of the oven for 25 minutes. Leave to cool in the tin.

4. For the filling, put margarine, sugar, syrup and condensed milk into a pan and stir over a gentle heat until the sugar dissolves. Bring to the boil and boil the mixture for 7 minutes, stirring continuously.

5. Remove pan from the heat, add vanilla essence and beat the mixture well. Pour the mixture onto the shortbread base, and leave to cool and set.

6. For the topping, roughly chop the chocolate and melt in bowl over pan of very hot water. Spread evenly over the filling. Leave to set, then cut into 16 squares.

"Every May half term we go camping near to Salcombe, Devon. I have been going since I was a baby, and now we take the girls. Milly and Bessie have fond memories of rock climbing there, and collecting seaglass with Daddy. When I was 8, I met my penpal Emma on the beach, and we still write to each other now. My mother got this flapjack recipe from Emma's parents and made it frequently when I was a child."

Hannah

Albert & Dawn's Flapjacks

YOU WILL NEED...

250g butter
600g oats
110g demerara sugar
1 tablespoon honey

MAKE IT!

1. Preheat the oven to 180°, 160° (fan), gas mark 4.
2. Melt the butter in a saucepan over a low heat and stir in the sugar and honey until the sugar has dissolved. Take off the heat and stir in the oats.
3. Put into a suitable baking tin – we use a 23cm square brownie tin. Bake for 10–14 minutes.
4. Leave to cool and cut into rectangles.

> **"The smell of shortbread always takes me back to Grandma's house, and I always have a smile on my face when I bake it, thinking back to how she always used to apologise, saying it wasn't 'up to her usual standard.'"**

Aunty Sarah

Grandma Dixon's Shortbread

YOU WILL NEED...

145g plain flour
30g semolina
115g butter
60g caster sugar
a pinch of salt

MAKE IT!

1. Preheat the oven to 170°, 160° (fan), gas mark 4.
2. Cream butter and sugar together, then add flour, semolina and salt and mix to form a soft dough.
3. Tear off a walnut-sized piece from the dough. Form into a small ball and put onto a lightly greased baking tray.
4. Press each ball with the back of a fork until flat and about 5cm across.
5. Bake for 20 minutes, remove from the oven and sprinkle with caster sugar.

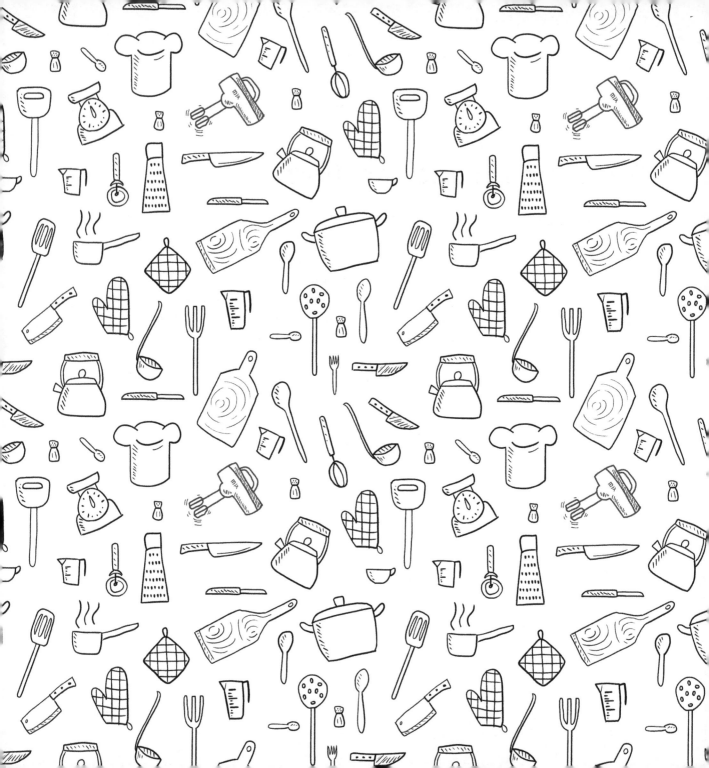

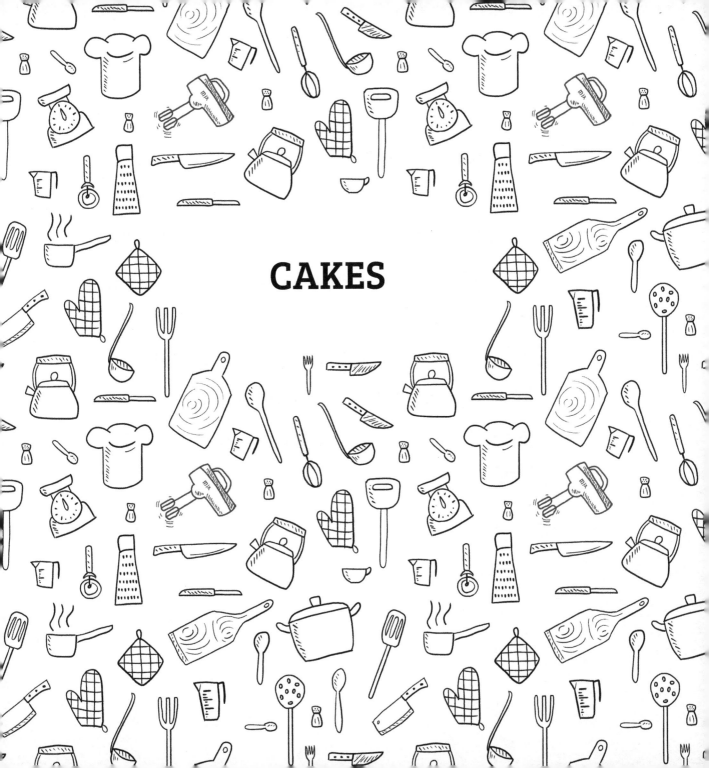

CAKES

"My mum always made this recipe if we had a family get-together, or when it was her birthday and she wanted to take cakes into work. Everybody loves it – everybody! Now I make it if we have people round or for parties. If I take it to work I always keep a piece out because by the time I get to the staff room there's only crumbs left!"

Rachel

Rachel's Polish Cake

... – as in the nationality, not furniture cleaner!

YOU WILL NEED...

125g butter
250g digestive biscuits
1 tablespoon golden syrup
2 desert spoons cocoa
    powder
150g chocolate

MAKE IT!

1. Melt the butter, golden syrup and cocoa powder in a pan on the stove.
2. Bash up the digestives (putting them in a bag and whacking them with a rolling pin is a good way to do this).
3. Mix the biscuits into the melted butter mixture and then put into a lined tin. Squash it down so it is pressed in firmly. Put into the fridge for a couple of hours.
4. Melt the chocolate in a bowl over boiling water and then spread on top of the biscuit mixture. Make patterns with a fork in the chocolate and then leave to set.
5. Cut it into small squares.

Bessie's Top Tip

Make sure you press the mixture into the tin *really firmly* so it doesn't crumble when you cut it.

59

"When my son Otto was born I made a new friend, Mandy, and we spent a lot of time meeting for cups of tea and cake. Mandy gave me this recipe – it looks impressive but is very easy to make. I always take it to our annual cousins' meet-up and it never lasts long!"

Cousin Harriet

Malteser Tray Bake

YOU WILL NEED...

100g of butter

3 tablespoons golden syrup

200g milk chocolate

400g digestive biscuits

175g Maltesers (plus extra
    for munching on while you
    make the tray bake)

200–300g white chocolate

MAKE IT!

1. Put the butter, syrup, and milk chocolate (hold back a few squares to decorate the top) in a pan and melt together on a gentle heat.

2. Crush the digestives as fine as possible (I use a food processor) and stir into the butter–chocolate mix. Once well mixed, add the Maltesers.

3. Lightly grease a small baking tray and line with grease-proof paper. Press the mixture firmly into the tray.

4. Melt the white chocolate in a bowl over a pan of simmering water, then pour onto the Malteser base and spread evenly. Finally, melt the last few squares of milk chocolate and pour over the white chocolate; use a toothpick to swirl the two chocolates together in a pretty marble pattern.

5. Put in the fridge to set for 1–2 hours. Cut into small pieces before it sets too hard.

Bessie's Top Tip

To save time I just dribbled the white chocolate onto the mix and didn't worry about marbling – it was much quicker and just as nice.

"OK – can a recipe get any easier (or tastier) than this? We found this in Aunty Wendy's cake book and I do remember my mother making it when I was young – I think she may have shoved some raisins in to make it feel less sinful – clearly concerned about our 5-a-day intake long before the government were.**"**

Hannah

Mars Bar Cake

YOU WILL NEED...
3 Mars bars
85g margarine or butter
85g Rice Krispies

MAKE IT!
1. Chop Mars bars into 1cm slices and melt with the butter over a low heat. Mix well.
2. Remove from heat and stir in the Krispies.
3. Pour into a 23 × 23cm brownie tin and squash down, then cool in fridge until you can resist no longer.

Bessie's Top Tip
You could melt some chocolate and dribble it over the top.

63

"We call these 'Auntie Nic's Raspberry Brownies' because she made them first, and Joseph and Luke would always ask her to make them for us. Last year Luke made some himself, and his Grandpa made the mistake of telling Auntie Nic that Luke's tasted better. Big Mistake!"

Amanda

Raspberry Brownies

YOU WILL NEED...

250g salted butter
400g light brown sugar
200g dark chocolate
100g milk chocolate
4 large eggs
140g plain flour
200g raspberries
60g cocoa powder

MAKE IT!

1. Preheat the oven to 180°, 160° (fan), gas mark 4. Melt butter, sugar and chocolate in a pan on a low heat.
2. Take off the heat and stir in the eggs, one at a time.
3. Sieve the flour and cocoa powder together and add to the mixture, along with half the raspberries.
4. Pour mixture into a square brownie tin and sprinkle the remaining raspberries on the top.
5. Place into the hot oven for about 30 minutes. Check with a skewer. Some like it squidgy (me), some like it more cakey; it's up to you.
6. Allow to cool a bit – if you can! – and serve with crème fraiche or ice-cream.

Bessie's Top Tip

When I made these, they were very squidgy after 30 minutes in the oven so you had to eat them with a fork! If you are not eating them straightway, you may want to leave them in the oven for an extra 5 minutes or so and do the skewer test.

"My daughter Aoife was allergy-tested when she was 5 months old and we found out that she was allergic to eggs and dairy. I spent the next couple of years trying dozens of different egg-free chocolate cake recipes until I found this gem. Aoife has since outgrown her dairy allergy but will likely be allergic to egg for the rest of her life. I'm hoping to bake her birthday cakes using this recipe for years to come."

Clodagh

Egg-free Chocolate Cake

YOU WILL NEED...

200g plain flour
200g caster sugar
4 tablespoons cocoa powder
1 teaspoon bicarbonate of
   soda
½ teaspoon salt
5 tablespoons vegetable oil
1 teaspoon vanilla extract
1 teaspoon distilled white
   vinegar
250ml water

MAKE IT!

1. Preheat oven to 180°, 160° (fan), gas mark 4. Lightly grease a 20cm round cake tin.
2. Sieve together the flour, sugar, cocoa, bicarbonate of soda and salt. Add the oil, vanilla, vinegar and water. Mix together until smooth.
3. Pour into prepared tin and bake for 45 minutes. Remove from oven and allow to cool.

Bessie's Top Tip

Double this mixture to make two cakes and put buttercream icing in the middle, or put into small cases to make cupcakes and reduce cooking time to about 15 minutes.

"When I was little this was my birthday cake of choice every year – I do like chocolate, and this is very chocolatey. I found a copy of the recipe in my Grandma's 1976 recipe book so we've been making it for a while. My bro (Uncle Sam) makes it every Christmas – he used to take it to his in-laws every year, but they prefer trifle so he would eat the whole thing on his own over a couple of days! Now Milly and Bess are happy to help him out (as am I – let's not pretend!)."

Hannah

Grandma Lesley's
Chocolate Refrigerator Cake

YOU WILL NEED...

110g unsalted butter

170g dark chocolate

200g rich tea biscuits, crushed (do not be tempted to swap and use digestive biscuits – they do not work!)

3 eggs, beaten

50g grapes, halved

2 tablespoons sherry

140ml double cream, lightly whipped

MAKE IT!

1. Melt butter and chocolate over low heat, then stir in the crushed biscuits.

2. Remove from heat and add the beaten eggs. Stir well to blend, then add the grapes and sherry.

3. Fold in cream. Put into a suitably sized cake tin and refrigerate for 3–4 hours.

Bessie's Top Tip

Decorate with squirty cream – if your mum will let you!

Hannah's Top Tip

Go for a long walk or wear stretchy trousers to enjoy this.

69

"It's now tradition for our friend Will to make this for us when we visit on Christmas Eve. It is very delicious. Caz, his mum, lets us add squirty cream to the bowl because, as she says, 'It *is* Christmas!'"

Bessie

Will's Christmas Chocolate Log

YOU WILL NEED...

3 eggs
75g caster sugar
55g self-raising flour
20g cocoa powder

1 small tub double cream
icing sugar (I usually add this
by eye and taste)

100g soft margarine or
unsalted butter
200g icing sugar
½ teaspoon vanilla essence
2 tablespoons cocoa powder

MAKE IT!

1. Grease and line a Swiss roll tin. Preheat the oven to 200°, 180° (fan), gas mark 6.
2. Whisk eggs and sugar using an electric whisk until thick and foamy (you should see the trail of the whisk and should be able to write your initials).
3. Sieve flour and cocoa mixture all over the top, then gently fold in the flour using a spatula or a palette knife.
4. Pour into the Swiss roll tin and tilt it gently to allow the mixture to flow to the corners. Bake for 10–15 minutes until springy to the touch.
5. Turn out onto a sheet of greaseproof paper, then quickly trim the edges to make a straight-sided rectangle. Roll up the Swiss roll and leave to cool on a rack.
6. For the filling, whisk the double cream, adding icing sugar to sweeten to taste. Whisk until spreadable.
7. Unroll the Swiss roll and spread the cream on the inside of the roll, leaving a 2cm clear area at the far end, and then roll back up again.
8. For the icing, cream together margarine or butter, icing sugar, vanilla essence and cocoa powder, then spread over the top of the log.
9. Add any decorations and serve.

"I love a really thick crumble topping whereas Aunty Jo likes a bit more fruit. This leads to endless debates in our house over the 'perfect' fruit-to-crumble ratio when we have crumble for our pudding. I absolutely need to have a huge dollop of really thick cream served with mine which makes it absolutely my favourite pudding. Cold crumble from the fridge served with milk the following day also makes a perfect breakfast!"

Jim

Uncle Jimmy's Apple Crumble

YOU WILL NEED...

500g apples, peeled,
   cored and sliced
1 teaspoon honey or sugar

175g plain flour
110g demerara sugar
110g butter

MAKE IT!

1. Put the apples in a pan and gently cook with 1 tablespoon of sugar or honey to soften them up a bit – about 10 minutes. Place in an oven-proof serving dish.

2. For the crumble topping, mix the sugar with the flour, then add the butter, cut into small pieces. Rub the butter into the flour and sugar mix with your fingertips.

3. Cook at 180°, 160° (fan), gas mark 4, for 30 to 40 minutes or until the topping is golden brown.

4. Serve with thick cream, custard or ice-cream (or all three!).

Bessie Top Tip

You can substitute some of the flour with porridge oats and sprinkle demerara sugar on the top to make a crunchier topping. We add blackberries to the apples as they grow in the allotment.

> **"This was my first foray beyond fairy cakes: I was having people for dinner and wanted to appear grown-up. It is completely idiot-proof, looks and tastes amazing and lends the baker an air of competence they may (or may not) possess."**

Julie

Julie Guppy's Favourite Upside-down Pear Cake

YOU WILL NEED...

200g butter, softened
75g light brown soft sugar
6 tablespoon raspberry
  liqueur (e.g. Chambord)
  – substitute with golden
  syrup for kids
4 conference pears, peeled,
  halved and cored
175g golden caster sugar
200g self-raising flour
3 medium eggs, beaten
4 tablespoon milk
custard, to serve

MAKE IT!

1. Heat the oven to 180°, 160° (fan), gas mark 4. Mash together 50g of the butter and the brown sugar using a fork, then mix in 4 tablespoon of the raspberry liqueur or syrup.
2. Spread onto the base of a deep, 23cm non-stick cake tin (if using syrup, line the cake tin with baking paper). Place on a baking tray as there will be a fair amount of leaking!
3. Press the pears, cut-side down, into the base.
4. Using an electric whisk, beat together the golden caster sugar, remaining butter, flour, eggs and milk until well blended. Spread over the pears.
5. Bake for 45–50 minutes until risen and firm to the touch. Leave to cool in the tin for 5 minutes, then turn out.
6. Drizzle over the remaining 2 tablespoon raspberry liqueur if using, then slice and serve warm with custard.

Bessie's Top Tip

Arrange the pears in a nice pattern or your mum will moan at you and tell you they look like pig trotters!

75

"I love making this because it is so delicious and easy. It also reminds me of our trip with Daddy and Babar to the Cheesecake Factory when we were on holiday in Florida – the slices there were HUGE!"

Milly

Milly's Nigella Cheesecake

INGREDIENTS

150g crumbled digestive
   biscuits

100g butter

340g cream cheese

300ml double cream

65g icing sugar

1 teaspoon vanilla essence

½ teaspoon lemon juice

1 jar of (expensive!)
   cherry jam

MAKE IT!

1. Put the biscuits in a large plastic bowl and bash them with a rolling pin until they are crumbled into small pieces and crumbs. Soften the butter and mix with the biscuit crumbs, then press into a 20cm loose-bottomed cake tin.

2. Blend the cream cheese, icing sugar, vanilla essence and lemon juice together until smooth.

3. Lightly whip the double cream and fold into the cream cheese mixture. Gently spoon this mixture on to the biscuit base and smooth with a spatula.

4. Place in fridge for at least three hours.

5. Just before serving, spread the cherry jam over the top.

Milly's Top Tip

I have also served this with fresh fruit on the top or with fresh fruit compote that our friend Julian made – that was delicious.

Hannah's Top Tip

This is based on Nigella Lawson's Cherry Cheesecake, but we have added extra base and increased the amount of cream cheese and cream so that we don't have annoyingly small amounts of leftovers.

"When we visited my Nana she always gave us a big batch of pies to put in the freezer. Sadly she was nearly blind and often put the wrong label on each pie. We never knew what we were getting until my mum cut into it at the dinner table! Luckily she only ever made sweet fillings..."

Sam

Nana's Surprise Pies

YOU WILL NEED...

225g unsalted butter, chilled
and cut into small chunks
375g plain flour
3 tablespoons caster sugar
80ml ice water

500g chopped rhubarb *or*
675g sliced apples *or*
900g plums, stoned *or*
450g sliced apples and
225g blackberries

MAKE IT!

1. Combine flour and sugar in a bowl. Add the butter and rub in with your fingertips until the mixture resembles breadcrumbs. Stir with a fork while you add the cold water until the dough starts to clump.

2. Lightly knead dough in the bowl until it forms a ball. Divide in two and flatten each portion into a disc. Chill for about 30 minutes.

3. Preheat the oven to 200°, 180° (fan), gas mark 6. Roll out the pastry discs and use one to line a shallow 23cm pie dish, ensuring the pastry overhangs the edge of the dish.

4. Put your chosen filling in the pastry-lined dish and sprinkle with caster sugar to taste. Use the other rolled-out pastry disc as a lid, pinching together the edges around the rim of the pie dish, then crimping them with a fork. Poke a small hole in the centre of the lid to allow steam to escape.

5. Brush with milk, sprinkle with a little caster sugar and cook for 40–50 minutes. Cover with aluminium foil during baking if the pastry starts to brown.

Bessie's Top Tip

We made a pie and took it to my cousins so they could play guess the pie (it was rhubarb!).

"This recipe is of a cake my mum used to make. We all loved it and I took the recipe. During lockdown, I made the cake for my granddaughters, who are 11 and 8. The older one loves it, but Isla, the younger one, thinks it is yuk! Nia, the elder one has now made it herself and even wants it for her birthday cake. It's really easy as you just put everything in together. If you like cinnamon it's very tasty!"

Susan

Susan's Speedy Spice Cake

(endorsed by the red kites of Watlington)

YOU WILL NEED...

115g self-raising flour
1 level teaspoon mixed spice
½ teaspoon cinnamon
140g soft brown sugar
115g butter or margarine
2 eggs
1 tablespoon milk

55g butter
85g icing sugar
1 tablespoon milk
50g dried fruit (sultanas,
    currants, glacé cherries)

MAKE IT!

1. Grease and line two 15cm cake tins.
2. Mix flour, spices, sugar, butter or margarine, eggs and milk together until well combined (about 2 minutes).
3. Divide the mixture between the two tins and bake at 190°, 170° (fan), gas mark 5, for about 25 minutes. Turn out of the tins and allow to cool.
4. For the filling, combine butter, icing sugar and milk until smooth. Stir in the dried fruit.
5. Sandwich the two cake layers together with filling and sprinkle with icing sugar.

Bessie's Top Tip

Don't eat this if there are red kites around! I made this when we went camping and it was quite funny – while we were eating it, a red kite flew down and tried to grab Tara's slice from out of her hand. It made her spill her cup of tea all over her son, but luckily she saved her cake!

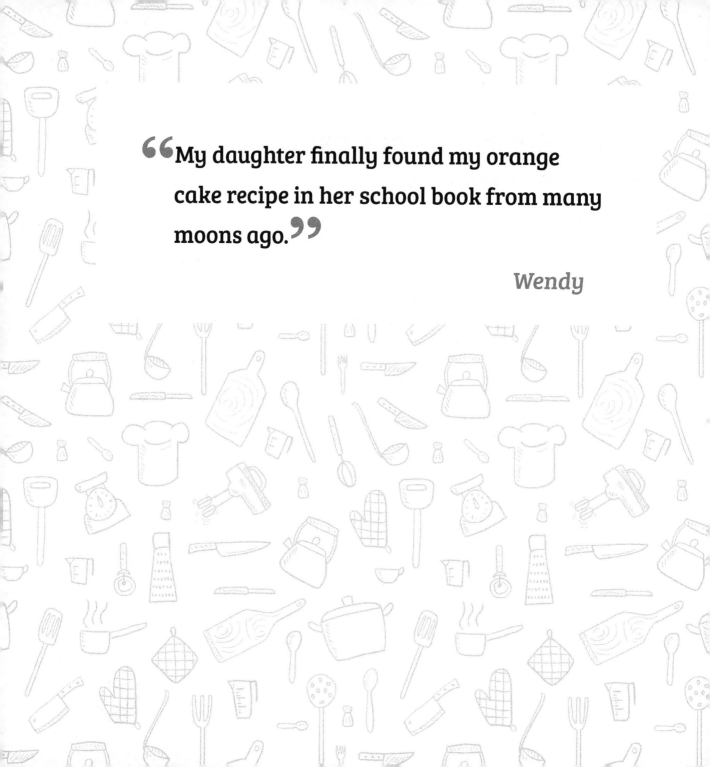

"My daughter finally found my orange cake recipe in her school book from many moons ago."

Wendy

Wendy Mitchell's Orange Cake

YOU WILL NEED...
125g self-raising flour
125g caster sugar
125g butter, softened, or
   block margarine
2 eggs
1 teaspoon baking powder
1 teaspoon vanilla essence
grated rind of an orange

MAKE IT!
1. Preheat the oven to 180°, 160° (fan), gas mark 4. Line a loaf tin with parchment paper.
2. Cream the butter and sugar together in a bowl until fluffy. Mix in the eggs, one by one.
3. Sieve flour and baking powder into the bowl and stir until well combined. Finally, stir in the vanilla and orange rind.
4. Pour into the prepared tin and bake for 40 minutes until it is, according to the illustrations,* 'nice and cakey'!

Bessie's Top Tip
Wendy's daughter's instructions are quite sparse so you could just throw all ingredients into the food mixer and see what happens (which was we did), or you can follow the method given above.

Use the orange – squeeze out the juice and stir in 3 tablespoons icing sugar, then poke holes in the cake with a skewer and drizzle over the glaze. It makes it really moist – delicious!

....
*   See inside back cover

83

"This recipe was always my favourite birthday cake when I was a girl. I copied it out when I was little and still have it but you can see how old it is by the state of the paper. It's an American recipe that my mum got when we lived in the Caribbean so the measurements are in cups."

Madeline

Carrot & Pineapple Cake

YOU WILL NEED...

1½ cups (200g) self-raising flour
1 cup (200g) sugar
1 teaspoon baking powder
1 teaspoon bicarbonate of soda
1 teaspoon cinnamon
½ teaspoon salt
⅔ cup (160ml) vegetable oil
2 eggs
1 cup (90g) grated carrot
½ cup (100g) pineapple chunks in syrup
1 teaspoon vanilla extract

85g cream cheese
1 tablespoon butter
1 teaspoon vanilla extract
2 cups (250g) sifted icing sugar

MAKE IT!

1. Preheat the oven to 180°, 160° (fan), gas mark 4. Grease a 23 × 23cm tin.
2. Sift all dry ingredients together.
3. Add oil, eggs, carrot, pineapple and vanilla and mix until combined.
4. Pour into the tin and bake for 35–40 minutes, then cool and remove from tin.
5. For the icing, beat cream cheese, butter and vanilla extract until light and fluffy, then beat in the icing sugar until well mixed and spreadable. Top the cake and serve.

Bessie's Top Tip

I really like the pineapple in this – it makes it a bit different.

"This is my favourite family recipe. It reminds me of my Nanny and Grandad. I love eating blondies with them – it makes me happy."

Mariella

Nanny Walls' Blondies

YOU WILL NEED...
175g butter
200g soft brown sugar
1 egg
200g plain flour
1 teaspoon vanilla extract
½ teaspoon salt
50g dark chocolate
100g white or milk chocolate

MAKE IT!
1. Preheat the oven to 180°, 160° (fan), gas mark 4.
2. Melt the butter in microwave. Put the sugar in a food mixer, add the melted butter and mix.
3. Allow to cool, then stir in the egg and vanilla. Sieve flour and salt and fold into the mixture.
4. Chop the chocolate and stir into the batter, then transfer into brownie tin. Smooth into the corners of the tin using back of spoon.
5. Bake in the oven for 20 minutes, until the top is set. Remove and leave to cool before removing the blondies from the tin.

Bessie's Top Tip
These were really popular at Mariella's and my coffee morning.

> **"**This was handed down to me 50 years ago by my husband's aunt and I have made it every Christmas since. It was originally a very old WI recipe – although I have adapted it by soaking all the fruit in a healthy amount of brandy overnight before making the cake.**"**

Liz

Julian's Aunty Nancy's Christmas Cake

YOU WILL NEED...

340g currants
110g raisins
340g sultanas
110g glacé cherries
brandy

225g flour
225g brown sugar
225g butter
rind and juice of 1 lemon
170g mixed peel
60g almonds or walnuts
70ml brandy
4 large eggs
¼ teaspoon nutmeg
1 pinch mace
1 pinch mixed spice
1 pinch salt

METHOD

1. Pre-soak all the fruit overnight in brandy.
2. Preheat the oven to 140°, 120° (fan), gas mark 1.
3. Line a 20cm cake tin with a double layer of greaseproof paper.
4. Sift flour, spices and salt. Beat butter to a cream in a mixing bowl. Add sugar and beat well.
5. Fold in two tablespoons of flour to prevent eggs and butter mixture curdling. Break in the eggs whole, one at a time, beating between each addition.
6. Mix together fruit, mixed peel, lemon rind and almonds, then add to the egg-and-butter mixture.
7. Add flour to this mixture and stir until all is well mixed and the fruit well distributed.
8. Add lemon juice and brandy and stir well. Scrape into the lined cake tin.
9. Place in the oven to cook for 4 hours, but start checking after 3½ hours. Remove when a skewer stuck in cake is removed moist but clean. Cool cake upside down in its tin on a wire rack.

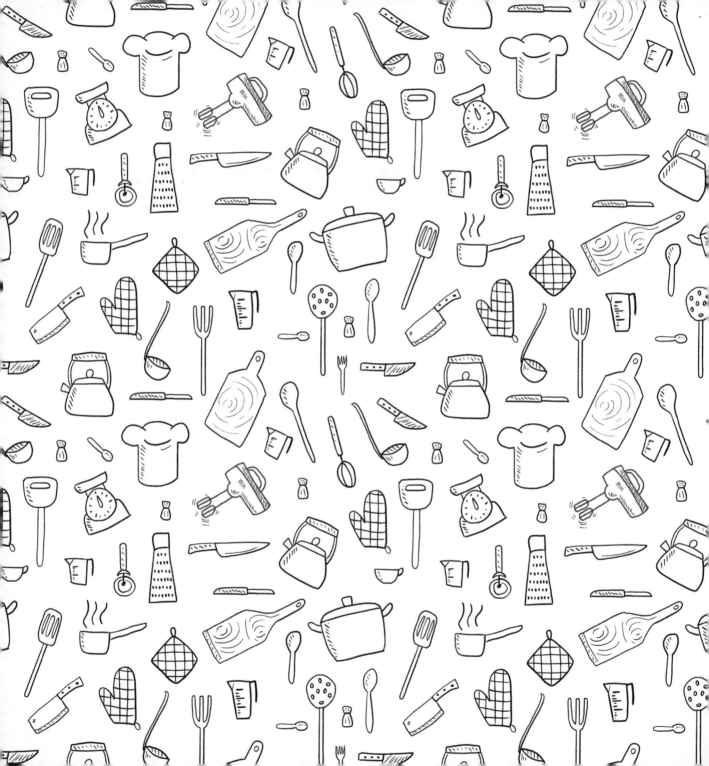

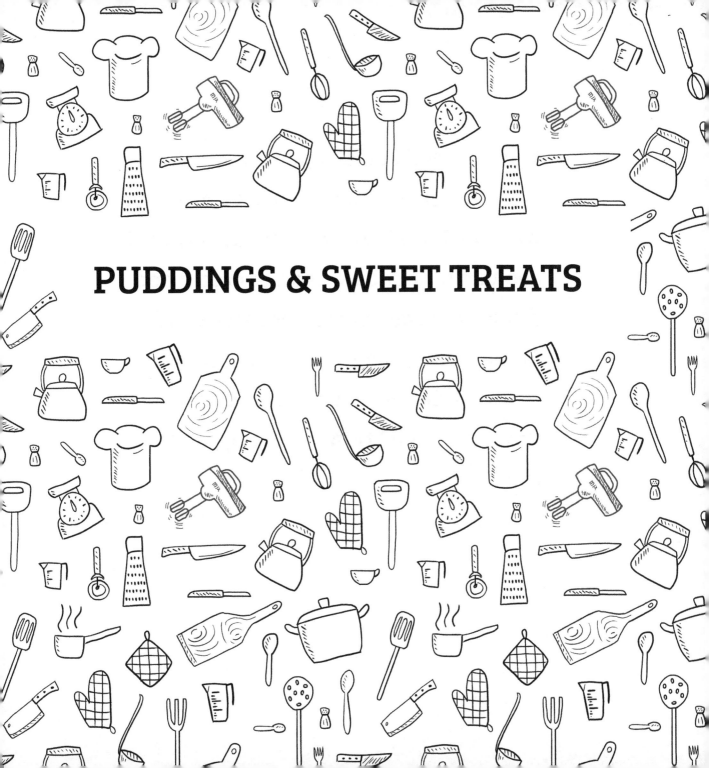

PUDDINGS & SWEET TREATS

"This is a really quick light dessert that was a family favourite when I was young. We often have fruit with low fat, natural yoghurt for pudding, but the cream and demerara sugar make this extra special. Aunty Wendy suggests using halved strawberries instead of the grapes in summer which I think is a very good idea."

Hannah

Grandma Joy's Grape Cream

YOU WILL NEED...

140ml double cream

140ml natural yoghurt

about 450g seedless grapes,
  halved

2 tablespoons demerara
  sugar

MAKE IT!

1. Mix the double cream with the natural yoghurt and put into large glass bowl. Stir in the grapes.

2. Chill in fridge. Sprinkle on the demerara sugar just before serving. There you are – a very quick and easy dessert!

"This recipe has been cobbled together from a number different recipes and has been made numerous times during lockdown. We don't have a very large freezer but we were really craving ice-cream. We decided to buy the ingredients and keep the milk and cream in the fridge until we had enough freezer space to put the ice-cream in! The great thing is that it's *so* easy to make, and it raised our spirits during lockdown."

Gerry

Eva & Lola's Easy-peasy Lockdown Oreo Ice-cream

YOU WILL NEED...

300ml double cream
300ml milk (whole or
   semi-skimmed is fine)
1 teaspoon vanilla essence
100g caster sugar
14 Oreo biscuits, finely
   ground

MAKE IT!

1. In a large, freezer-proof bowl add the cream, milk, vanilla and sugar and stir until the sugar has dissolved, then whisk with an electric mixer until the top is covered in bubbles. Freeze for one hour.

2. After an hour, remove the bowl, whisk again until the ice crystals have been broken down, then return to the freezer.

3. Repeat after another hour; the mixture should be starting to freeze now. At this point add the ground Oreos and mix well.

4. Refreeze and mix every hour for another 3–4 hours, depending on freezer temperature.

5. Once frozen, just cover and leave until you're ready to eat. This is also nice without Oreos as vanilla ice-cream, or melt 100g dark chocolate with the milk, cool and add to the remaining ingredients for a rich chocolate ice-cream.

Bessie's Top Tip

I set a timer so I would remember to keep whisking.

95

> **"I used to make this with my Grandma every Christmas Eve when I was little, and now I feel it's not a proper Christmas without a trifle."**
>
> *Holly*

Grandma Argument's Christmas Trifle

YOU WILL NEED...

1 packet of Boudoir biscuits
  (sponge fingers)
several good slugs of sherry
  (optional)
1 tin of fruit cocktail
1 packet of strawberry or
  raspberry jelly
1 tub of pre-made fresh
  custard
500g double cream
topping of your choice

MAKE IT!

1. Place halved sponge fingers into the bottom of a glass bowl and pour on the sherry, or the syrup or juice from the fruit cocktail if you're going down the non-alcoholic route. Allow the biscuits to soak up the liquid.

2. Spoon the fruit cocktail mix evenly over the sponge fingers.

3. Make the jelly as per the packet instructions; once cool, pour over the sponge and fruit. Leave in the fridge to set for 4 hours or ideally overnight.

4. Add the custard evenly on top of the jelly layer and return to the fridge while you whip the double cream into stiff peaks.

5. Use a fork to spread the cream on top of the custard, then decorate with your chosen toppings.

Bessie's Top Tip

I decorated with hundreds-and-thousands as the colours looked so pretty. You could use grated chocolate instead, or maybe fresh strawberries.

"I remember begging my mummy for this every day, and very rarely she would let me and Milly make it. We would have so much fun making it, but even more fun talking and drinking outside with the warmth of the sun (while Mummy cleared up all the mess!). Milly doesn't even like bananas, but she loves this."

Bessie

Lockdown Chocolate Banana Smoothie

YOU WILL NEED...

1 handful of ice
3 tablespoons of hot
　　chocolate powder
1 banana
1 tablespoon of honey

MAKE IT!

1. Put all the ingredients in a smoothie blender and mix until combined. Or use a stick blender and be very careful with your fingers.
2. Pour in a glass and enjoy!

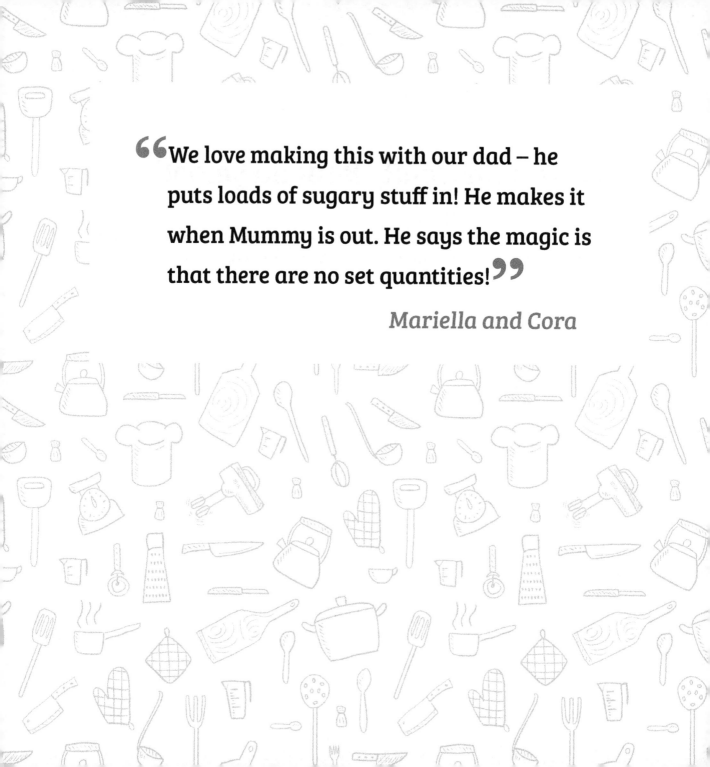

"We love making this with our dad – he puts loads of sugary stuff in! He makes it when Mummy is out. He says the magic is that there are no set quantities!"

Mariella and Cora

Owen's Fat Shake

YOU WILL NEED...
2 bananas
loads of ice-cream
double cream
a handful of chocolate,
    chopped
meringues

MAKE IT!
1. Put the bananas in the blender. Add equal amounts of vanilla ice-cream and double cream and blend until smooth.
2. Chop or smash some chocolate and hand-crush a few meringues and stir into the ice-cream mixture.
3. Put in the freezer for 3 minutes, then stir and pour.

Hannah's Top Tip
Beware! This recipe comes with a health warning from Mariella's mother Julie – apparently it's way too sweet...

101

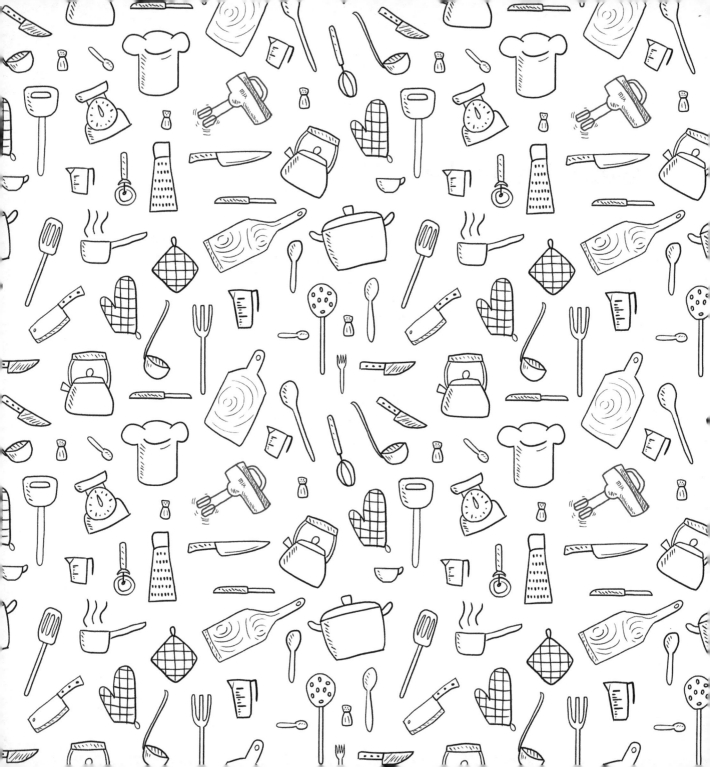

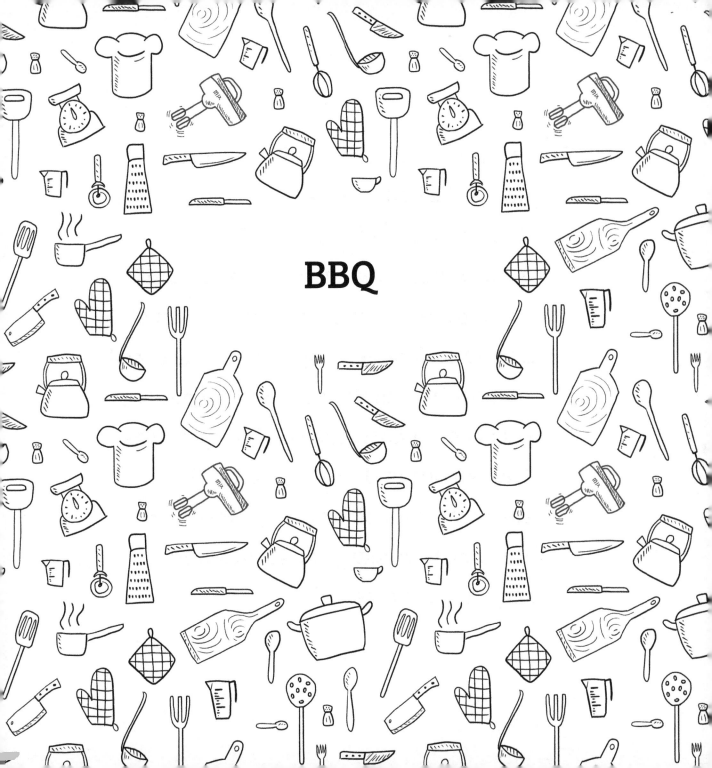

BBQ

"We had a huge barbecue in our back garden. We had to poke the woodpile with a broom to check for snakes. Mostly we cooked Aussie beef sausages on it, but if new or posh guests visited, Mum would use it to cook honey soy chicken and sliced potatoes. Inevitably the chicken would be well beyond chargrilled and the potatoes black outside and raw inside. I still remember the look on Aunty Margaret's face as she politely gnawed on Mum's incinerated efforts."

Emma

Mum's 'Impress Aunty Margaret' Honey Soy Chicken

YOU WILL NEED...

4 chicken breast halves
3 tablespoons soy sauce
3 tablespoons honey
1 teaspoon ground ginger
1 teaspoon crushed garlic

MAKE IT!

1. In a plastic container, make the marinade by combining soy sauce, honey, ginger and garlic.
2. Add the chicken halves, seal the container and shake until chicken is fully coated. Chill for 4 hours or overnight.
3. To cook, place pieces of chicken on barbecue (once the flames have died down, to avoid my mum's mistake). Turn once, pouring or brushing on a little of the leftover marinade if desired.
4. Cook for about 10 minutes until tender, but no longer pink.

"Campfires are a memory of nearly every holiday I went on growing up in Australia. Often someone would appear with a bag of flour and whip up some damper. Sometimes someone would even rustle up a billy (a tin can with a loop of wire for a handle) and make billy tea. This is Aussie campfire tucker from the time of Australia's first British settlers."

Emma

Campfire Damper

YOU WILL NEED...

2 cups (240g) self-raising
   flour
a pinch of salt
2 teaspoons sugar (optional)
2 tablespoons butter
¾ cup (175ml) milk
8 long, clean sticks

MAKE IT!

1. Combine flour, salt and sugar in a bowl. Rub in butter until resembling breadcrumbs.
2. Gradually add milk and stir with a knife to make a dough.
3. Divide into 8 pieces. Stretch each piece of dough into a snake and twist onto a stick.
4. Hold over campfire embers, turning regularly, for 10 minutes or until golden brown.

Bessie's Top Tip

Emma made some damper for us when we went camping with her – it was delicious dipped into jam.

Billy Tea

YOU WILL NEED...

1 litre water
2 gum leaves
about 3 tablespoons black
   loose leaf tea

MAKE IT!

1. Build tripod with branches and suspend billy from it over the campfire. Bring water to the boil.
2. Add the tea and gum leaves and set aside for 5 minutes to steep.
3. Swing billy back and forth to get tea leaves to sink (or strain if you want to avoid scalds!). Serve black and hot.

Bessie's Top Tip

Not sure where you are going to find gum leaves – so maybe just use the hot water for hot chocolate instead?

"Bessie and her sister Milly have been members of Elfins (Woodcraft Folk) for years and loved that their dad used to help out. At the weekend camp one year they made cakes in hollowed-out oranges – they loved getting messy scooping out the orange and eating it before filling it with the cake mixture. This is perhaps the only time I would approve of using a packet of cake mix – you are not going to want to measure out ingredients in the middle of a windy field!"

Hannah

Elfin Campfire Cake Orange

YOU WILL NEED...

10 oranges
prepared cake batter mix
   from a packet
aluminium foil

MAKE IT!

1. Cut the top of the oranges to make a lid and spoon out the inside (eat this if you want!).

2. Pour batter mix inside the orange up to ¾ full and replace the top.

3. Wrap in foil and carefully place into the smouldering embers of the fire. Avoid the flames and cook for approximately 30 minutes, turning the oranges at least once.

"Do we need to give instructions for these? According to Milly, Bessie and friends, no BBQ or camping trip would be authentic without the toasting of marshmallows at the end so we include this for the sake of completeness. There are several variations of course but this is how we do it – mainly because Neil has a strong chocolate digestive habit so we always have a ready supply."

Hannah

Easy S'mores

YOU WILL NEED...

1 packet of chocolate
   digestives
1 large packet of
   marshmallows
skewers or toasting forks

MAKE IT!

1. Once the fire or BBQ coals are glowing nicely, skewer a marshmallow on the end of a stick or toasting fork and toast gently over the fire. (The reality is that the kids will plunge it straight in and wait until it catches fire 'cos it's fun.)

2. Once it's nicely golden (or black!) on the outside, manoeuvre the marshmallow between two chocolate digestives, with the chocolate on the inside. Squidge it a bit to melt the chocolate.

3. Eat and repeat!

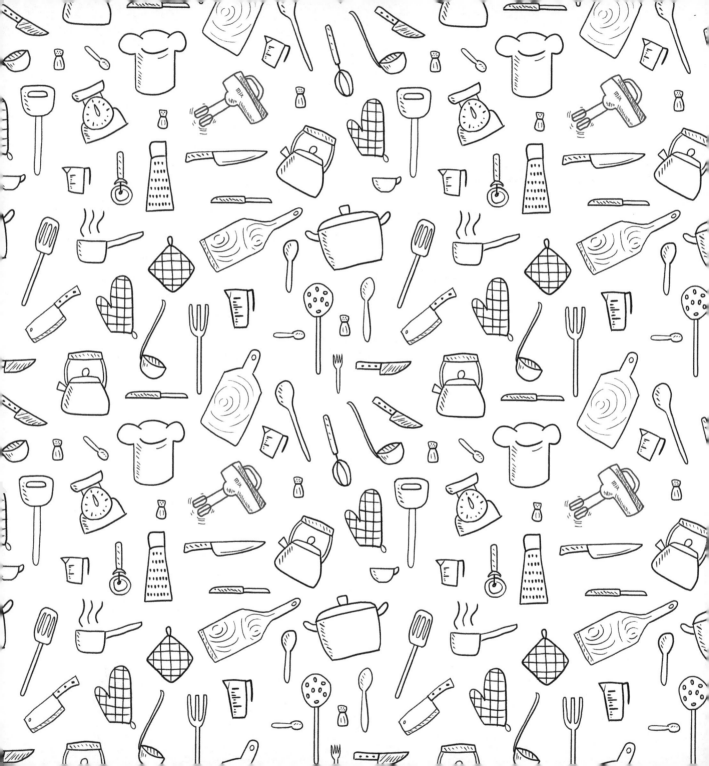

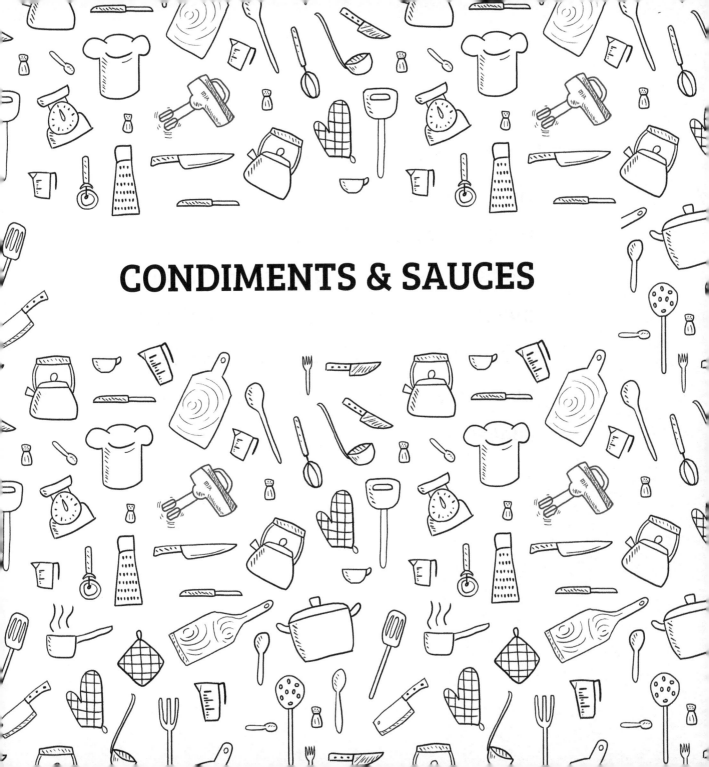

CONDIMENTS & SAUCES

"The only time Grandpa got a look-in in the kitchen was chutney-making season, towards the end of the summer. He grew a lot of tomatoes, and I have an abiding memory of them left to ripen on all the windowsills of their house. I guess he made this chutney when they ran out of space!"

Hannah

Grandpa Dixon's Green Tomato Chutney

YOU WILL NEED...

2.25kg green tomatoes
450g onions
10g peppercorns
25g salt
450g sugar
1l vinegar
225g raisins
225g sultanas

MAKE IT!

1. Slice the tomatoes, chop the onions and mix together in a basin with the peppercorns and salt. Allow to stand overnight.
2. The next day, boil the sugar in the vinegar, then add the raisins and the sultanas. Simmer for 5 minutes then add the tomatoes and onions and continue to simmer until thick.
3. Pour into sterilised jars (see Step 1 on p.117).

Bessie's Top Tip
My dad loves this in his cheese and ham sandwiches.

"Shirley is a prolific jam and pickle maker – likely as a result of her husband's abundant vegetable and fruit garden. She has been supplying me ever since I shared a house with her daughter Amanda in 1995. Bessie and Milly are always grateful recipients of her jams; Neil prefers her pickles and chutneys."

Hannah

Shirley Brain's Jumbleberry Jam

INGREDIENTS

equal amounts of mixed soft
  berries and sugar (500g of
  each makes about two jars)
a squeeze of lemon juice

MAKE IT!

1. Place clean jam jars into the oven on a low heat. Put a couple of saucers in the freezer.

2. Put the fruit and sugar into a high-sided saucepan. Over a medium heat, stir to dissolve the sugar completely.

3. Add the lemon juice and bring to a rolling boil. Boil until set – this can take up to 20 minutes (but see Bessie's Top Tip below).

4. To test, put some jam on a saucer from the freezer and wait for a 10 seconds or so to cool. If it wrinkles when you push it with your finger, it's ready. Pour into the hot sterilised jars and seal.

Bessie's Top Tip

Don't let this boil for too long – I accidentally made Blackberry Concrete and had to throw the jam away, which was a shame as we had collected the blackberries from our allotment.

"When we go camping, our friend Jo always does 'platas frutas' – a massive plate of mixed chopped fruit. When Aunty Emma sent me the recipe for this sauce I knew it would go perfectly with platas frutas – and it did!"

Bessie

Gooey Caramel Sauce

YOU WILL NEED...

100g light brown sugar
100g butter
100ml cream or milk
   (either is fine)

MAKE IT!

1. Put the butter and sugar in a saucepan over a low heat until the butter has melted and the sugar has dissolved, but not burned.
2. Add the cream or milk and heat until bubbling, stirring continually. Take off the heat and leave to cool for few minutes before serving.

Bessie's Top Tip

This is perfect on ice-cream too. Keep leftovers in an airtight jar in the fridge – then you can have it the next day too.

"This is a very flexible recipe and we never measure the ingredients so sometimes it's really chewy and other times it's not. Either way it is delicious and much better than the fake chocolate sauce you get in plastic bottles – trust me!"

Bessie

Grandma Lesley's Chocolate Sauce for Ice-cream

YOU WILL NEED...
6 squares of dark chocolate
large knob of butter
about 2 tablespoons golden
   syrup

MAKE IT!
1. Put the chocolate into a saucepan over a low heat until it has nearly melted, then add the butter and stir until it melts.
2. Add the syrup and stir for a minute. Pour over ice-cream.

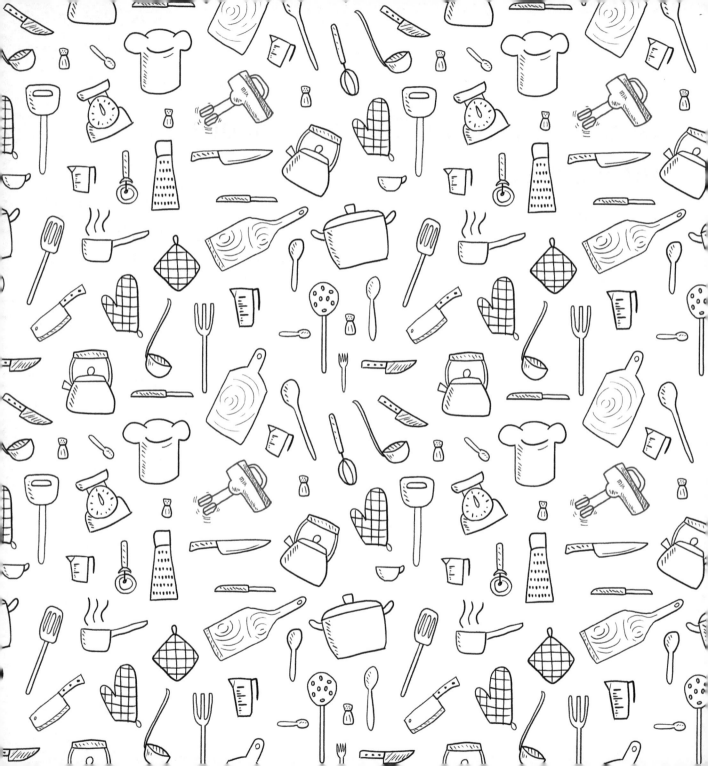

Acknowledgements

Ever since Neil's diagnosis we have been overwhelmed by the help and support we have received from family and friends; frankly, that is what has got us through some tough times.

Bringing up children when one parent has a diagnosis of dementia is no simple task, and it would be very easy for Milly and Bessie to feel like passive witnesses to their father's illness. Instead we have encouraged them to learn and talk about Alzheimer's and, in doing so, have inspired them to raise money and help others. This book seemed like a natural progression from the memory walks, tabletop sales and coffee mornings they have already done.

The cliché that it takes a village to raise a child rings true for me: I am eternally grateful to everyone who has got on board with this project and helped Bessie and me create this book.

Thank you to everyone who replied to our request and contributed a recipe, and apologies to anyone whose recipe we weren't able to include.

Thank you to everyone who helped us sample the various bakes over the summer – without you we would be the size of elephants by now!

Thank you to Caroline Gratrix, who kindly took the photos.

Thank you to Ian Guppy of Feelgood Creative for his work on the cover design.

Thank you especially to Anke Ueberberg and Matthew Flynn, who encouraged us and offered their expertise, not to mention a massive amount of time to get this book published.

And finally, thank you to everyone reading this who has purchased a copy – you're a star!

Engage with dementia and find support

Neil and I are both firm believers that a dementia diagnosis is nothing to be ashamed of; it is a disease like any other and we have always been open and honest about it.

I would urge anyone wondering about the behaviour of a loved one – or even their own – to contact their GP. Get the ball rolling with the local memory clinic and find out as much as you can. As scary as a diagnosis may appear, it is much better to know what you are dealing with. The earlier dementia is diagnosed, the more effective medication may be. You have time to gather information, access support and sort out legal matters.

One of the ways in which I have engaged with Neil's diagnosis was to become involved with Dementia UK. I now sit on their Lived Experience Advisory Panel (LEAP). We help Dementia UK remain relevant to the people they are supporting, offer feedback and help spread the word about Admiral Nurses.

As part of the panel I have met some fantastic people – carers, people living with a diagnosis, and professionals working in the field of dementia – and we invited a number of them to contribute a recipe. Bessie's favourites were from George and Wendy, who are living with a diagnosis of dementia, and Susan, whose husband has dementia.

George is co-chair of LEAP and writes a blog about living with dementia. He is an amazing example and advocate for people living with the disease: he thrives on being involved and improving the situation for all, so he was keen to support Bessie.

Susan's husband is now being cared for in a care home, and during the first lockdown she was unable to visit him. She found this very hard but channelled her upset and frustration into walking over 900 miles to raise money for Dementia UK. She also entertained us with her coronavirus-inspired lockdown poems.

I first heard Wendy speak at a dementia conference in Birmingham in 2016. I was still reeling from Neil's diagnosis and was seeking information to try and make sense of the situation. I attended the event to gather knowledge especially about young onset dementia.* Wendy's talk was inspirational – I had been thinking in terms of what had been taken from Neil, and here was Wendy showing how much was possible and could still be achieved despite a diagnosis of dementia. It was a real insight into how Neil may have been feeling – something that he found very hard to articulate.

A dementia diagnosis is tough. Neil, Milly, Bessie and I are fortunate that friends, family and the support of an Admiral Nurse have helped us keep mainly on an even keel. Not everyone living with dementia is as lucky, so we hope the funds raised by this book for Dementia UK will help to train more Admiral Nurses to support those who need them.

....

* Young onset dementia is defined as a diagnosis with dementia under the age of 65.

In aid of

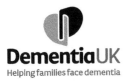

DementiaUK
Helping families face dementia

Dementia UK provides specialist dementia support for families through our Admiral Nurse service. When things get challenging or difficult for people with dementia and their families, Admiral Nurses work alongside them, giving them compassionate one-to-one support, expert guidance and practical solutions that can be difficult to find elsewhere. They are a lifeline – helping families to live more positively with dementia in the present, and to face the challenges of tomorrow with more confidence and less fear.

The Admiral Nurse Dementia Helpline is for anyone with a question or concern about dementia, including Alzheimer's disease. From looking out for the first symptoms of Alzheimer's to understanding the challenges of living with someone with vascular dementia, our specialist Admiral Nurses have the knowledge and experience to understand the situation and suggest answers.

You can call the Helpline for free on 0800 888 6678
or email helpline@dementiauk.org.

The Helpline is open 9am–9pm Monday to Friday
and 9am–5pm on Saturday and Sunday.

www.dementiauk.org

Dementia UK is a registered charity in England and Wales (1039404) and Scotland (SCO47429)

Lightning Source UK Ltd.
Milton Keynes UK
UKHW020833190421
382245UK00008B/553